Herbal
HEALTH

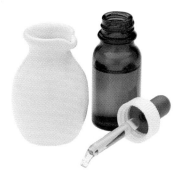

"He causeth the grass to grow for the cattle and herbs for the service of humanity"

Psalm 104:14

Herbal
HEALTH

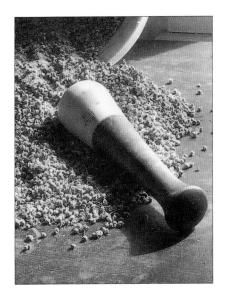

BRENDA LITTLE

A LOTHIAN BOOK

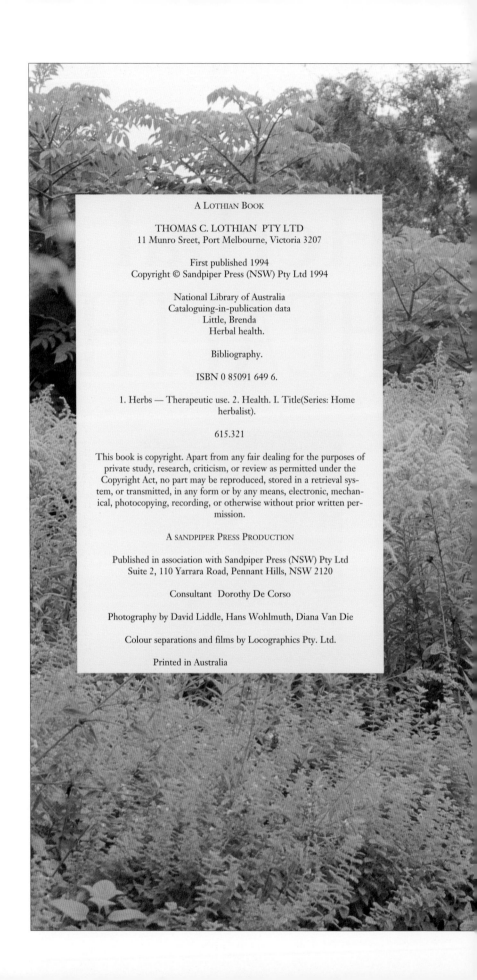

A Lothian Book

THOMAS C. LOTHIAN PTY LTD
11 Munro Sreet, Port Melbourne, Victoria 3207

First published 1994
Copyright © Sandpiper Press (NSW) Pty Ltd 1994

National Library of Australia
Cataloguing-in-publication data
Little, Brenda
Herbal health.

Bibliography.

ISBN 0 85091 649 6.

1. Herbs — Therapeutic use. 2. Health. I. Title(Series: Home
herbalist).

615.321

A SANDPIPER PRESS PRODUCTION

Published in association with Sandpiper Press (NSW) Pty Ltd
Suite 2, 110 Yarrara Road, Pennant Hills, NSW 2120

Consultant Dorothy De Corso

Photography by David Liddle, Hans Wohlmuth, Diana Van Die

Colour separations and films by Locographics Pty. Ltd.

Printed in Australia

Contents

INTRODUCTION

Introduction

It is not widely appreciated that before the present century when the powerful petroleum and chemical industries began to take charge of our way of life, the only medicines used came from plants.

Man had garnered knowledge of plant properties over the centuries. Knowledge had not come easily or quickly—it had been a case of trial and error, with possible death the likely result of error. Observation had been the tool which honed his skill.

The Chinese and Indian cultures accumulated medicinal plant knowledge which the Arabs of the ninth century, the Greeks and Romans and the European botanists of the Renaissance refined and expanded. The knowledge we have of the "green healers" comes to us down the centuries, validated by time and experience and more recently by scientific research.

The synthetic drugs we use today which have largely replaced the natural medicines have their advantages—and also their drawbacks. They can be effective in controlling the disease for which they are prescribed but the patient can develop a different drug-induced malady.

The plants our forefathers used to cure themselves are still around, their properties have not changed, they are still simple to grow and simple to use. They will promote our health and well-being and rescue us from irritating small ailments. Serious illness should of course be referred to professionals.

There was a time, not so very long ago, when anyone promoting herbal cures was thought to be a bit odd, or "way-out". That attitude has changed. In so many different ways we have found that Nature knows best and we are at last showing the respect due. Two hundred years ago Linnaeus said "What we know of the Divine Works are much fewer than of those of which we are ignorant". He is still right.

It is estimated that there are at least half a million

species of plant in the world and it comes as a considerable shock to learn that we have, as yet, only identified about ten per cent of their organic constituents. Fortunately science is showing greater interest in medical botany these days with ignorance being reduced quickly as a result.

Growing medicinal herbs is simple. There is no need to go to the lengths of having a "physick" garden as the monks of old used to—a few chosen plants tucked in among the flowers and vegetables or grown in tubs will be little trouble. Enthusiasm may make you want to establish a herb garden. Herbs are not fussy plants so labour and upkeep will be minimal.

Drying, storing and using herbs demand little expertise and present no problems. The whole enterprise can be very enjoyable and the rewards most pleasing.

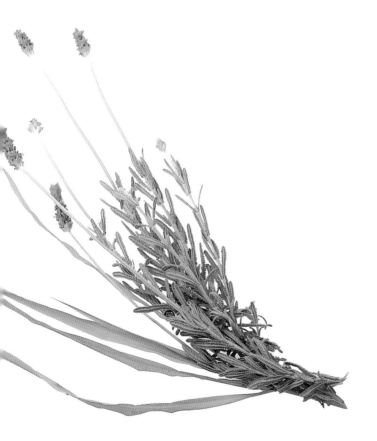

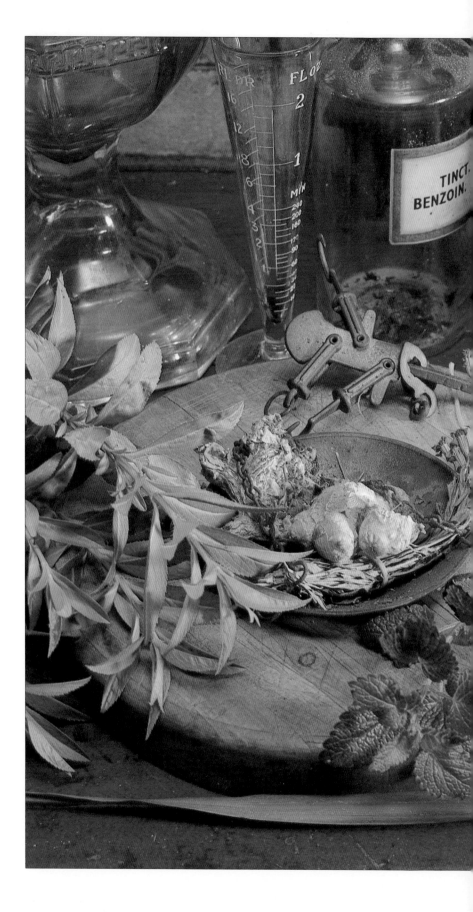

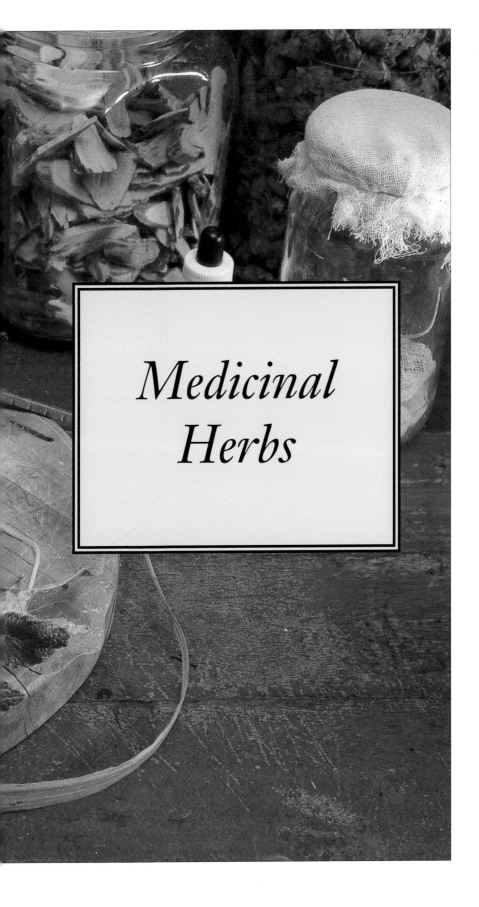

Medicinal Herbs

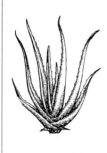

ALOE

Aloe vera

Parts used
The thick gel found in the leaves

Every kitchen should have a potted aloe plant. That way it is easy to cut off the thick, fleshy leaves and squeeze the clear gel onto an injury.

Arab traders carried aloe from Spain to Asia around the 6th century and used it to treat skin problems. But it was the Chinese who developed similar uses used in the West.

Contemporary herbalists use aloe in some of the same ways the Greek physician Dioscorides used it almost 2,000 years ago—externally for burns and wounds.

Applications

WOUNDS, BURNS, SCALDS, SCRAPES, SUN-BURN, DRY SKIN, FUNGAL INFECTIONS AND INSECT BITES

Gel
To help soothe wounds, burns, scalds, and sunburn, and to help avoid infection, select a lower (older) leaf, cut several centimetres off, slice it lengthwise, apply the gel, and allow it to dry. Clean the wound properly with soap and water first.

A perfect house-plant, aloe requires little water and no special care.
It prefers sun, but will tolerate shade and doesn't mind poor soil.
It requires good drainage and temperatures above 4 degrees C (40 degrees F).

Ointment
Cut the leaves and collect a large quantity of gel then boil it down to a thick paste. Store in a cool place and use as the fresh leaves.

Tonic
Mix 2 tsp of gel with a glass of water or fruit juice. Take three times a day.

Inhalation
Use the gel in a steam inhalation for bronchial relief.

Caution
High internal doses of the leaves can cause vomiting.

ANGELICA

Angelica spp.

Parts used

Roots, leaves—leaves from *A. archangelica*; roots from *A. archangelica* and *A. senensis*

During the 17th century, angelica was a popular treatment for colds and respiratory ailments. When the colonists arrived in North America, they found many Indian tribes also using the herb to treat respiratory ailments, particularly tuberculosis.

Applications

RESPIRATORY AILMENTS, DIGESTIVE AID, ARTHRITIS, LIVER FUNCTION, ANAEMIA, MEN-STRUAL IRREGULARITIES

Tincture

Make from the leaves of *A. archangelica*. Take up to 3 ml three times a day for colds, flu, bronchitis, and asthma. A tincture from the root of *A. archangelica* is good for catarrh and chesty coughs.

Infusion

Use 1 tspn of powdered seeds or leaves per cup of boiling water. Steep 10 to 20 minutes.

An infusion of the leaves of *A. archangelica* taken in standard doses to help the digestion.

Compress

Make a compress and soak in a hot diluted tincture from the root of *A. archangelica* and apply to painful joints for arthritis.

Essential oil

Mix 10 drops of angelica oil in 25 ml of sunflower oil and massage arthritic or rheumatic joints.

Decoction

Use 1 tspn of powdered roots per cup of water. Bring to a boil and simmer 2 minutes. Let stand 15 minutes. Make a decoction from the root of *A. senensis* and take for liver stagnation, anaemia and menstrual irregularities.

Caution Fresh angelica roots are poisonous. Drying eliminates the hazard. Herb gardeners should be sure to dry angelica roots thoroughly before using them.

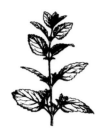

LEMON BALM

Melissa officinalis

Parts used
Leaves

Bees love this fragrant herb, which explains its generic name, melissa— Greek for "bee."
The ancient Greek physician Dioscorides applied balm leaves to skin wounds and added the herb to wine to treat a variety of illnesses. The Roman naturalist Pliny recommended it to stop bleeding. During the 10th century, Arab doctors recommended balm for nervousness and anxiety.

Medieval Europeans also used balm for nervousness and anxiety. Melissa water, or Eau de Melisse, was a popular tranquillizer and sedative.

Balm contains chemicals (polyphenols) that help fight several infection-causing bacteria as well as eugenol, an anesthetic, that helps relieve wound pain.

Applications

DEPRESSION, TENSION, SWELLINGS, SORES, INSECT BITES, DIGESTION

Compress
Make a hot compress using 2 teaspoons of leaves per cup of water. Boil 10 minutes, strain, and apply with a clean cloth to relieve painful swellings.

A relaxing bath
Tie a handful of balm in a cloth and run your bathwater over it. In addition to feeling its tranquil effect, you'll love its lemony aroma.

To treat wounds
To help treat a minor cut, crush some fresh balm leaves and apply them directly to the wound.

Tincture
In a tincture, use half to one and a half teaspoons up to three times a day. Best made from fresh leaves. It has a similar action to the infusion but is stronger.

has a similar action to the infusion but is stronger.

Infusion

For a light, lemony-tasting infusion, to help soothe the stomach, fight infection, nervous exhaustion and depression or ease menstrual pain, use 2 teaspoons of leaves per cup of water. Steep 10 to 20 minutes. Drink up to 3 cups a day.

Ointment

For sores and insect bites.

Infused oil

Use warm as a gentle massage oil to help relieve tension and depression.

Balm grows to 30cm with small, two-lipped, white or yellow flowers, which bloom in bunches throughout the summer. The above-ground parts die back each winter, but the root is perennial.

Balm likes well-drained soil with a pH near neutral. The herb prefers partial shade. It wilts in full sun and loses some aroma.

For medicinal use, the leaves should be harvested before the plant flowers. Cut the entire plant a few centimetres above the ground. Dry it quickly or the leaves may turn black. Balm loses much of its fragrance when dried. After drying, powder the leaves, then store them in tightly sealed opaque containers to preserve the volatile oil.

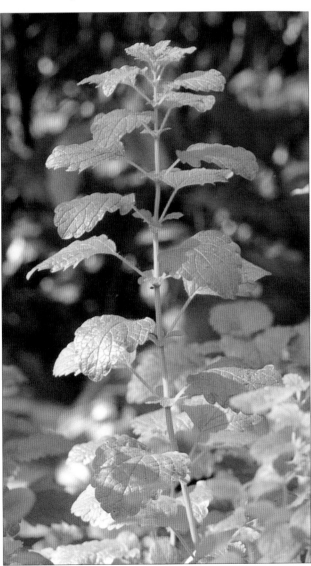

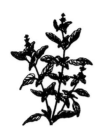

BASIL

Ocimum basilicum

Parts used
Leaves

In India, basil has long been revered as a sacred herb. The native species is even called *Ocimum sanctum*, "holy basil."

Basil's reputation in healing has been mixed. The ancient Greek physician Dioscorides and the influential Roman doctor Galen both warned against taking basil internally, saying it caused insanity and spontaneous generation of internal worms.

But the Roman naturalist Pliny and Arab physicians 1,000 years later defended it as a great healer, as did the Chinese, who used it to treat stomach, kidney, and blood ailments.

Applications

ACNE, DEPRESSION, ITCHING SKIN

Infusion
For an infusion, use 2 to 3 teaspoons of dried leaves per cup of boiling water. Steep 10 to 20 minutes. Apply with a cotton ball to treat acne. Indian researchers have reported that basil kills bacteria when applied to the skin. They have used basil oil successfully to treat acne.

Tincture
Use half to 1 teaspoon up to three times a day.

Fresh leaves
Rub on insect bites to reduce inflammation and itching.

Essential oil
Add about 10 drops to a hot bath for nervous exhaustion or mental fatigue.

Caution
Basil should not be given in medicinal quantities to children under age 2.

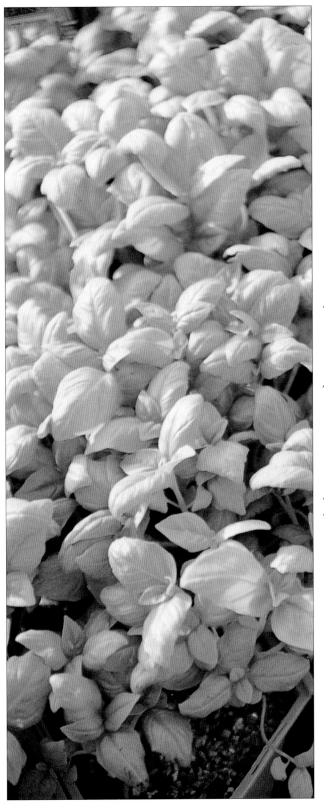

An aromatic annual that reaches 60cm, basil has spikes of small white or purplish flowers that blossom in summer.

Basil grows best in well-drained, manure—or compost-amended soil under full sun.

Pinching promotes bushiness. After six weeks, cut the main stem above a node to produce twin-stem plants. Trim branches every few weeks. Use fresh leaves, or dry and store them in airtight opaque containers.

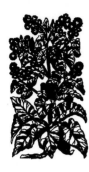

BURDOCK

Arctium lappa

Parts used
Leaves, root, seeds

Burdock—the name is a combination of bur, from its tenacious burrs, and dock, Old English for "plant"—seems to reach out and grab anything that comes near it.

Early Chinese physicians considered burdock a remedy for colds, flu, throat infections, and pneumonia. India's traditional Ayurvedic healers used it similarly.

Later European herbalists prescribed burdock root for fever, cancer, eczema, psoriasis, acne, dandruff, gout, ringworm, skin infections, syphilis, gonorrhea, and problems associated with childbirth.

Contemporary herbalists recommend it for skin problems, wound treatment, urinary tract infection, arthritis, sciatica, ulcers, and even anorexia nervosa. German researchers have discovered fresh burdock root contains chemicals (polyacetylenes) that kill disease-causing bacteria and fungi.

Applications

SKIN DISORDERS, SORES, BOILS, FUNGAL SKIN INFECTIONS

Decoction
For a decoction, boil 1 teaspoon of root in 3 cups of water for 30 minutes. Cool. Drink up to 3 cups a day. It has a sweet taste similar to celery root.

Use for skin disorders, especially boils, sores and dry skin.

Also use the decoction as a wash for acne and fungal skin infections such as athlete's foot.

Poultice
Apply a poultice from the root to skin sores and ulcers. A poultice of leaves can be applied to bruises and skin inflammations.

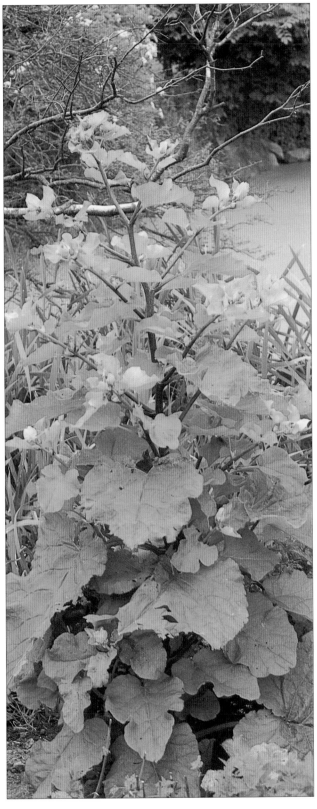

Burdock's medicinal root has brown bark and a white, spongy, fibrous interior, which becomes hard when dried. Its stem is multi-branched, with long, egg-shaped leaves. Each branch is topped by a bristled "flower," actually a clump of many purplish flowers, which produces its infamous burrs.

Burdock prefers moist, rich, deeply cultivated soil and full sun but tolerates poorer soils.

Harvest the roots during the autumn of the first year or the spring of the second.

CELERY

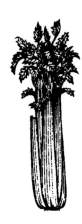

Apium graveolens

Parts used
Seeds, root, stalk

Scientists have discovered a surprising number of healing benefits in celery seed. They help relieve insomnia and high blood pressure

India's traditional Ayurvedic physicians have prescribed celery seed since ancient times as a diuretic to treat water retention and as a treatment for colds, flu, indigestion, arthritis, and diseases of the liver and spleen.

Contemporary herbalists recommend celery as a diuretic, tranquillizer, sedative, and menstruation promoter, and as treatment for gout, arthritis, obesity and anxiety.

Applications

ARTHRITIS, HYPERTENSION, URINARY DISORDERS

Infusion
Try a pleasant-tasting infusion as a mild relaxant or to bring on menstruation. Use 1 to 2 teaspoons of freshly crushed seeds per cup of boiling water. Steep 10 to 20 minutes. Drink up to 3 cups a day.
An infusion of 1 teaspoon of crushed seeds to per cup of boiling water will clear the acid from joints relieving arthritic symptoms and gout.

Tincture
In a tincture, using seeds as in the infusion, take half to 1 teaspoon up to three times a day to relieve urinary tract infections.

A tincture from the root has been used in the past as a diuretic for hypertension and urinary disorders.

Essential oil
Dilute 10 drops in about 20 ml of sunflower oil and massage arthritic joints.

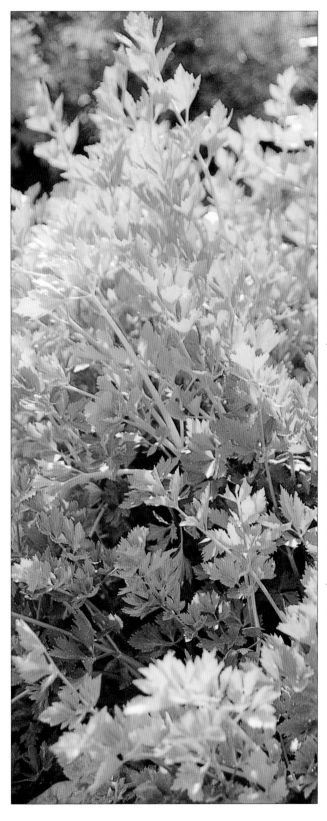

Celery grows best in well-watered, richly organic soil. Less ideal conditions produce tougher, stringier, more bitter stalks.

In mild areas, celery grows virtually year-round. Soak seeds before planting. Germination typically takes about ten days. Transplant when seedlings are about 7cm high at approximately three months. Space plants about 15cm apart.

Water copiously. Stalk juiciness depends on how much water the plants receive.

Harvest seeds when they mature.

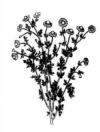

CHAMOMILE

Chamaemelum nobile & Matricaria recutita

Parts used
Flowers

Chamomile is not one herb, but two—German (or Hungarian) chamomile and Roman (or English) chamomile. The two plants are botanically unrelated, but they both produce the same light blue oil used in healing since ancient times.

The Greek physician Dioscorides and the Roman naturalist Pliny recommended chamomile to treat headaches and kidney, liver, and bladder problems India's ancient Ayurvedic physicians used it similarly.

Germans have used chamomile since the dawn of history for digestive upsets and as a menstruation promoter and treatment for menstrual cramps.

Contemporary herbalists recommend chamomile externally to spur wound healing and treat inflammation, and internally for fever, digestive upsets, anxiety, and insomnia.

Applications

INSOMNIA, ANXIETY, STRESS, TENSION, IRRITABLE BOWEL SYNDROME, INSECT BITES, STRAINED EYES, HAY FEVER, BRONCHITIS, MOUTH INFLAMMATIONS

Bath
For a relaxing bath, tie a handful of chamomile flowers into a cloth and run your bathwater over it.

The herb depresses the central nervous system; when you feel anxious take a hot "chamomile" bath.

Infusion
For a refreshing infusion, use 2 to 3 heaped teaspoons of flowers per cup of boiling water. Steep 10 to 20 minutes.

Drink a cup at night for insomnia, anxiety or stress. Also take for irritable bowel syndrome.

Use as a mouthwash for any ulcers or inflammations.

For cuts, scrapes, or burns, brew a strong infusion, cool it, and apply in compresses.

Tincture
Will have the same benefits as the infusion.

In a tincture, use half to 1 teaspoon up to three times a day.

Dissolve 5-10 drops of tincture in warm water for use as an eyewash to treat strained eyes.

Inhalation
Add 2 teaspoons of flowers to boiling water and inhale for hay fever or bronchitis.

Essential oil
Chamomile oil applied to the skin reduces the time it takes burns to heal.

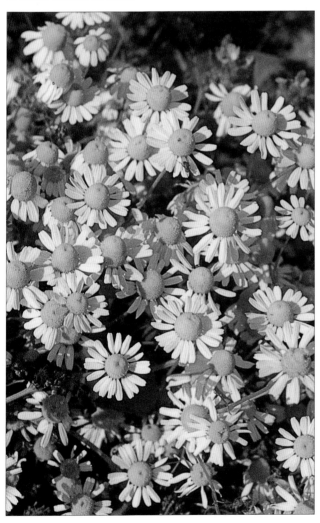

German chamomile is an annual that reaches 90cm. The Roman herb is a perennial groundcover that rarely exceeds 22cm. Both have downy stems, feathery leaves, and daisy-like flowers with yellow centers and white rays.

German chamomile prefers sandy, well-drained soil in partially shaded gardens. It flowers at about six weeks.

Perennial Roman chamomile double-flower variety, preferred by herbalists, adapts to almost any soil but favours moist, well-manured loam.

Roman chamomile does best when it's stepped on. Walking on it releases the herb's lovely fragrance and does not hurt the plant.

After harvesting, dry the flowers and store them in sealed containers to preserve their volatile oil.

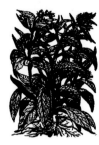

COMFREY

Symphytum officinale

Parts used
Roots, leaves

The early Greeks first used comfrey root external-ly to treat wounds, believing it encouraged torn flesh to grow back together. The Roman naturalist Pliny "verified" this practice with the observation that boiling comfrey in water produces a sticky paste capable of binding chunks of meat together.

Comfrey paste hardens like plaster, and cloths soaked in it were often wrapped around broken bones on ancient battlefields. When the paste dried, the result was a primitive but effective cast. This treatment earned comfrey the popular names "knit-bone" and "boneset".

Comfrey contains a chemical (allantoin) which encourages cartilage, bone and muscle cells to grow. When the herb is crushed and applied to an injured limb the allantoin is absorbed through the skin speeding up the healing proccess.

Be sure to wash wounds thoroughly with soap and water before applying comfrey or the rapid heal-ing process may trap dirt and infection.

Applications

MINOR FRACTURES, BONE OR MUSCLE DAM-AGE, BRUISES, SPRAINS

For wound treatment, comfrey roots are preferable to the leaves. Roots contain more than twice as much allantoin.

*Caution
This herb has restricted usage in Australia and New Zealand.
 Do not use this herb internally.*

Poultice
Puree the leaves and apply to minor fractures not set in plaster—broken toes, ribs etc.

Infused oil
Use for arthritic joints, bruises and sprains.

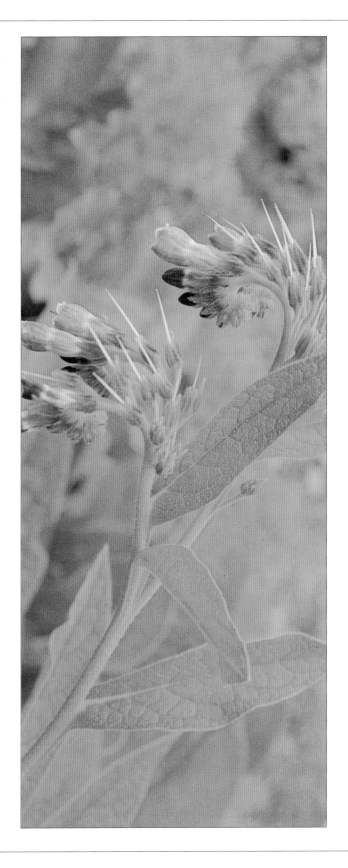

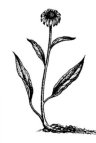

CONEFLOWER, PURPLE

Echinacea spp.

Parts used
Root

Coneflower was the American Plains Indians' primary medicine. They applied root poultices to all manner of wounds, insect bites and stings, and snakebites. They used it as a mouthwash for painful teeth and gums and drank it as tea to treat colds, smallpox, measles, mumps, and arthritis.

In 1870, a patent-medicine purveyor, Dr. H. C. F. Meyer of Nebraska, used it in his Meyer's Blood Purifier. He promoted the remedy as "an absolute cure" for rattlesnake bite, blood poisoning, and a host of other ills.

Contemporary herbalists are enthusiastic about coneflower for its antifungal and antibacterial properties. The herb contains a natural antibiotic (echinacoside), which is comparable to penicillin in that it has broad-spectrum activity.

Applications

INFECTION, INFLAMMATION, COMMON CATARRH AND COLDS, FOOD POISONING, SNAKE BITE, SORE THROAT, WOUNDS

Decoction
Use to take advantage of coneflower's infection-fighting potential or as a possible treatment for arthritis.

To make a decoction, bring 2 teaspoons of root material per cup of water to a boil, then simmer 15 minutes. Take 10ml doses every 2-3 hours for acute infections.

Bathe the infected area around wounds.

Tincture
In a tincture, take 2-5ml doses every 2-3 hours for chills and colds. Take in 10ml doses for snake bite and food poisoning.

Gargle 10ml in a glass of warm water for a sore throat.

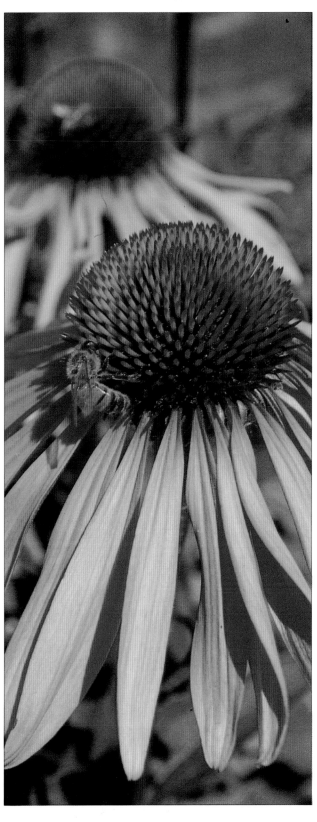

Coneflower is a 60-150cm perennial whose flowers resemble black-eyed susan, with purple rays radiating from a cone-shaped center—hence its common name, purple coneflower. Coneflower has black roots, a single stem covered with bristly hairs, and narrow leaves. Coneflower grows from seeds or root cuttings taken in spring.

Don't cover seeds—tap them into moist, sandy soil.

Coneflower grows in poor, rocky, slightly acidic soil under full sun, but it also thrives in richer soils.

It takes three or four years for roots to grow large enough to harvest.

Harvest the roots after flowering; wash, chop and dry.

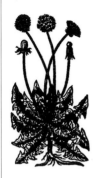

DANDELION

Taraxacum officinale

Parts used
Leaves, root

Chinese physicians have prescribed dandelion since ancient times to treat colds, bronchitis, pneumonia, hepatitis, boils, ulcers, obesity, dental problems, itching, and internal injuries.

Tenth-century Arab physicians were the first to recognize that dandelion increases urine production. Contemporary herbalists recommend dandelion leaves almost exclusively as a diuretic for weight loss, premenstrual syndrome, menstrual discomforts, swollen feet and high blood pressure.

Applications

DIURETIC, CLEANSER, WARTS

Fresh stalks
The sap from the fresh plant can be effective against warts. Apply directly from the stem or the root.

Infusion
For a leaf infusion, use 14g of dried leaves per cup of boiling water. Steep 10 minutes. Drink 3 cups a day. Use for cleansing toxic conditions and as a digestive stimulant.

Tincture
For a root decoction, gently boil 2 to 3 teaspoons of powdered root per cup of water for 15 minutes. Cool. Drink up to 3 cups a day.

Take 1 to 2 teaspoons up to 3 times a day.
Use for toxic conditions such as acne and eczema.

Diuretic
Diuretics can help eliminate water weight, but should not be used for permanent weight control.

The diuretic may also help relieve the bloated feeling of premenstrual syndrome.

If you're using dandelion leaves as a diuretic (for premenstrual syndrome or high blood pressure) or digestive aid, take it as a root decoction, or tincture. The taste is reasonably pleasant.

Diuretics deplete the body of potassium, an essential nutrient. People taking diuretics should be sure to eat foods high in potassium, such as bananas and fresh vegetables.

Fortunately, dandelion causes no potassium loss than other diuretics because the herb itself is high in potassium.

Caution

Dandelion may cause skin rash in sensitive persons.

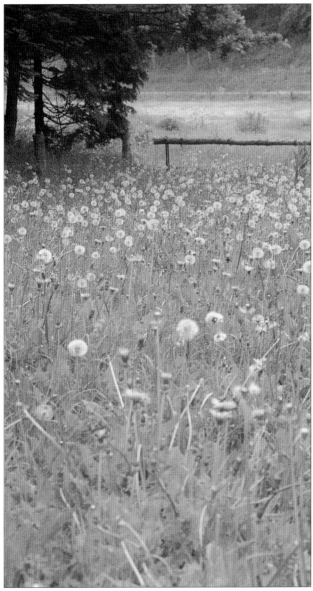

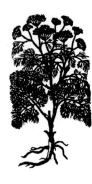

FENNEL

Foeniculum officinale

Parts used
Seeds, root

During the third century B.C., Hippocrates prescribed fennel to treat infant colic. Four hundred years later, Dioscorides called it an appetite suppressant and recommended the seeds to nursing mothers to boost milk production.

The Roman naturalist Pliny included fennel in 22 remedies. He noted that some snakes rubbed against the plant after shedding their skins and soon after, their glazed eyes cleared. Pliny took this as a sign that fennel cured human eye problems, including blindness.

By the 17th century, fennel was a mainstay of herbal healing.

Contemporary herbalists recommend fennel as a digestive aid, milk promoter, expectorant, eyewash, and buffer in herbal laxative blends.

Applications

DIGESTIVE AID, GUM DISORDERS, SORE THROAT, NERVOUS STOMACH

Seeds
As a digestive aid, chew a handful of seeds.

Infusion
Caution Avoid high doses during pregnancy. Fennel seeds are safe, but fennel oil may cause skin rash in sensitive individuals.

To make a pleasant, licorice-flavored infusion, use 1 to 2 teaspoons of bruised seeds per cup of boiling water. Steep 10 minutes. Drink up to 3 cups a day.

Take for indigestion, acidity, colic or griping pains. It has a carminative action.

Tincture
In a tincture, take half to 1 teaspoon up to three times a day.

Like most other aromatic herbs, fennel appears to relax the smooth muscle lining of the digestive tract (making it an antispasmodic).

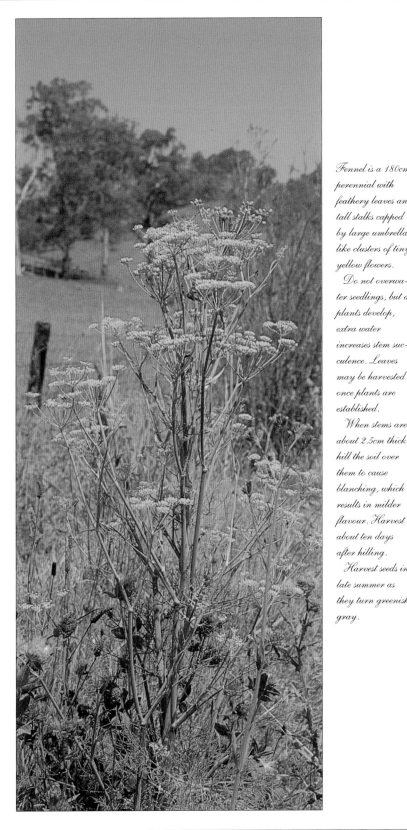

Fennel is a 180cm perennial with feathery leaves and tall stalks capped by large umbrella-like clusters of tiny yellow flowers.

Do not overwater seedlings, but as plants develop, extra water increases stem succulence. Leaves may be harvested once plants are established.

When stems are about 2.5cm thick, hill the soil over them to cause blanching, which results in milder flavour. Harvest about ten days after hilling.

Harvest seeds in late summer as they turn greenish gray.

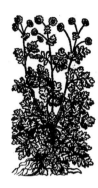

FEVERFEW

Tanacetum parthenium

Parts used
Leaves

During the Middle Ages, the Greek name for the herb, parthenion faded, and the plant was renamed featherfoil because of its feathery leaf borders. Featherfoil eventually became feverfew.

Once feverfew acquired its name, herbalists decided it was a fever treatment.

Some herbalists recommended feverfew for other ailments, particularly headache.

Applications

MIGRAINE HEADACHES, PERIOD PAIN

Fresh leaves

In the 1970s the wife of the chief medical officer of Britain's National Coal Board suffered chronic migraines. A miner heard about her problem and told her he'd also been a long-time migraine sufferer—until he started chewing a few feverfew leaves every day. The woman tried the herb, noticed immediate improvement, and after 14 months was free of her searing headaches.

For migraine control, chew two fresh (or frozen) leaves a day, or take a pill or capsule containing 85 milligrams of leaf material. If feverfew capsules do not provide benefit after a few weeks, don't give up on the herb without changing brands. "Feverfew" pills and capsules contain only trace amounts of the herb.

Tincture

Take 5-10 drops every 30 minutes at before a migraine. Feverfew is a prophylactic. You take the remedy daily in order to prevent migraine attacks.

Infusion

Use half to 1 teaspoon per cup of boiling water. Steep 5 to 10 minutes. Drink up to 2 cups a day.

Take feverfew in the form of an infusion to help lower blood pressure, as a digestive aid, or to help bring on menstruation.

Caution

Chewing the leaves can give you mouth ulcers.

If you are taking any kind of blood thinning drug avoid feverfew.

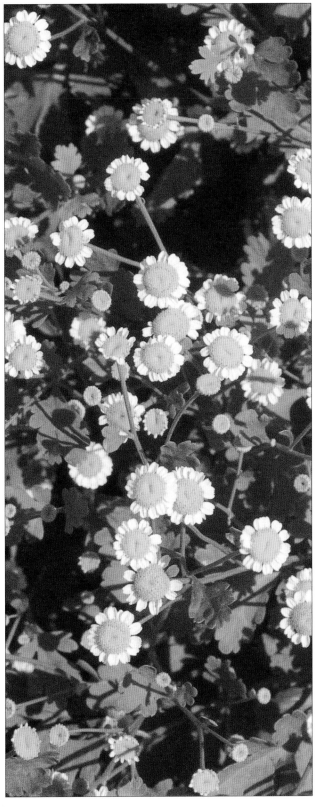

Feverfew is a perennial that reaches 90cm and has daisy-like flowers with yellow centers.

Feverfew does best in partial shade. Compost stimulates better growth. Pinch back flower buds to encourage bushiness.

Harvest leaves when they become mature.

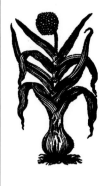

GARLIC

Allium sativum

Parts used
Bulb

Garlic appeared prominently in the world's old-est surviving medical text, the Ebers Papyrus. It was an ingredient in 22 remedies for headache, insect and scorpion bites, menstrual discomforts, intestinal worms, tumors, and heart problems.

The Greek physician Hippocrates recommended it for infections, wounds, cancer, leprosy, and digestive problems. And Pliny listed it in 61 remedies for ailments.

During World War I, British, French, and Russian army physicians treated infected battle wounds with garlic juice. They also prescribed garlic to prevent and treat amoebic dysentery.

Applications

WARTS, HIGH CHOLESTEROL, DIGESTIVE DISORDERS, CORNS, FUNGAL INFECTIONS, HIGH BLOOD PRESSURE, SKIN INFECTIONS, CHEST PROBLEMS

Infusion
For an infusion, chop six cloves per cup of cool water and steep 6 hours.

Tincture
For a tincture, soak 1 cup of crushed cloves per quart of brandy, shake daily for two weeks, then take up to 3 tablespoons a day.

Fresh cloves
One medium-size garlic clove packs the antibacterial punch of about 100,000 units of penicillin. Depending on the type of infection, oral penicillin doses typically range from 600,000 to 1.2 million units. The equivalent in garlic would be about 6 to 12 cloves. It's best to chew 3 cloves at a time, two to four times a day.

Rub fresh onto acne and mash to use on warts.

To help reduce blood pressure and cholesterol, three to ten cloves of fresh garlic a day is recommended.

Garlic must be chewed, chopped, bruised, or crushed to transform its medicinally inert alliin into antibiotic allicin.

Caution

Garlic may irritate the stomach.

To eliminate garlic breath, try chewing traditional herbal breath fresheners: parsley, fennel, or fenugreek.

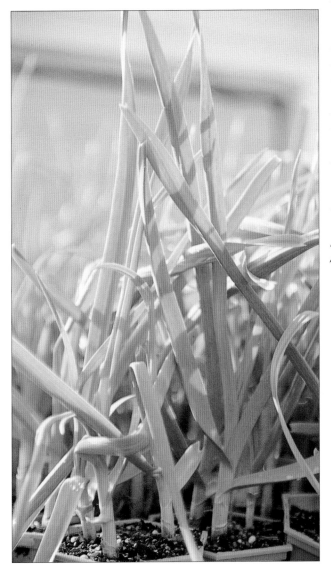

Garlic grows easily from cloves. Plant them 5cm deep and 15cm apart.

Garlic thrives best in rich, deeply cultivated, well-drained soil. Do not overwater. Full sun produces the largest bulbs, but garlic tolerates some shade.

During summer, cut back the flower stalks so the plant devotes all its energy to producing fat, aromatic bulbs.

Harvest bulbs in late summer. Store them in cool darkness.

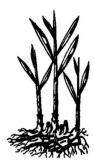

GINGER

Zingiber officinalis

Parts used
Roots

Ginger appeared prominently in China's first great herbal, the Pen Tsao Ching (Classic of Herbs), compiled by Shen Nung around 3000 B.C. Shen Nung recommended ginger for colds, fever, chills, tetanus, and leprosy.

Chinese sailors began chewing ginger to prevent seasickness, and Chinese physicians prescribed it to treat arthritis and kidney problems. Chinese women still drink ginger tea for menstrual cramps, morning sickness, and other gynecological problems.

They also consider ginger an antidote to shellfish poisoning, which is why Chinese fish and seafood dishes are often seasoned with the herb.

Applications

MOTION SICKNESS, NAUSEA, MORNING SICK-NESS, DIGESTIVE AID, COLDS

Capsules
For motion sickness, the recommended dose is 1,500 milligrams 30 minutes before travel. Commercial ginger capsules are usually most convenient.
Also used for morning sickness.

Tea
Use tea as a digestive aid; to help treat colds and flu, nausea, morning sickness, or arthritis. To make ginger tea, use 2 teaspoons of powdered or grated root per cup of boiling water. Steep 10 minutes.

Caution
Be careful when using in pregnancy, although it can be taken safely for morning sickness in the doses described.

Tincture
2-10 drops a dose for nausea, indigestion and menstrual cramps.

Decoction
For colds and flu add 1-2 slices of fresh ginger to a cup of water and simmer for 10 minutes.

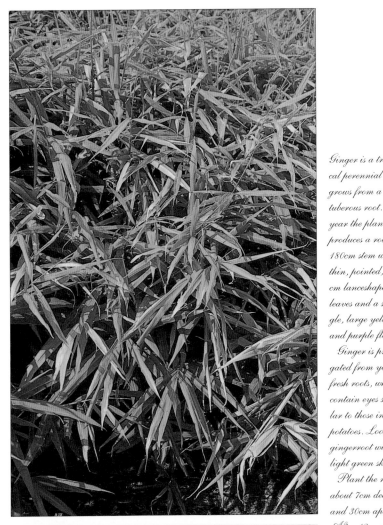

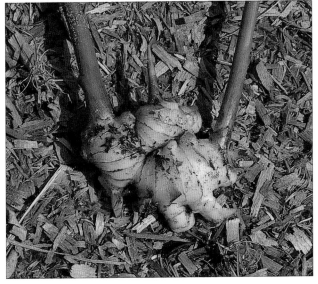

Ginger is a tropical perennial that grows from a tuberous root. Each year the plant produces a round, 180cm stem with thin, pointed, 15 cm lanceshaped leaves and a single, large yellow and purple flower.

Ginger is propagated from young fresh roots, which contain eyes similar to those in potatoes. Look for gingerroot with light green skin.

Plant the roots about 7cm deep and 30cm apart. After 12 months, uproot the plant, harvest some roots, and replant the rest.

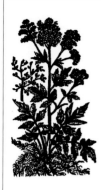

MARSHMALLOW

Althaea officinalis

Parts used
Root or leaves

Marshmallow was a food before it was a medicine.

The plant's history as a healer goes back to Hippocrates, who prescribed a decoction of marshmallow roots to treat bruises and blood loss from wounds. Four hundred years later, the Greek physician Dioscorides recommended marshmallow root poultices for insect bites and stings and prescribed the decoction for toothache and vomiting and as an antidote to poisons.

Tenth-century Arab physicians used mallow leaf poultices to treat inflammations.

The spongy material in marsh mallow roots is called mucilage. When it comes in contact with water, it swells and forms a gel.

Applications

CUTS AND WOUNDS, RESPIRATORY SYSTEM, IMMUNE SYSTEM, CUTS, SCRAPES, BURNS, GASTRITIS, PEPTIC ULCERS

Gel
To prepare for external use, chop the root very fine and add enough water to make a gooey gel. Apply the gel directly to superficial wounds, cuts, scrapes or sunburn.

Decoction
Enjoy a sweet decoction to take advantage of marshmallow's soothing potential and possible infection-fighting abilities. To make a decoction, gently boil half to 1 teaspoon of chopped or crushed root per cup of water for 10 to 15 minutes. Drink up to 3 cups a day.

Taken internally, it helps relieve upset stomach and the respiratory rawness associated with sore throat, cough, colds, flu, and bronchitis.

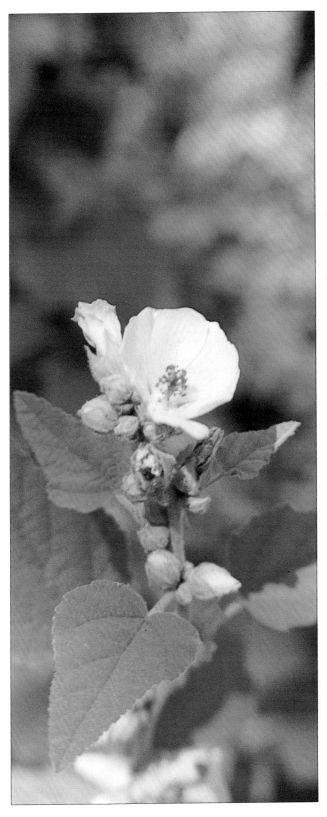

Marshmallow is a downy perennial with a long tap-root. The stems, which die back each autumn, are hairy and branching. The gray-green leaves, 3cm long, are toothed, and covered with velvety hairs. The flowers, pink or white, bloom in summer and give rise to round fruits called "cheeses," one of the herb's names.

In moist soil, under full sun, marshmallow is a hardy plant that grows easily from seeds, cuttings, or root divisions.

Do not harvest roots from plants less than two years old. In autumn, when the top growth has died back, dig out mature roots and remove the lateral rootlets. Wash, peel, and dry them whole or in slices.

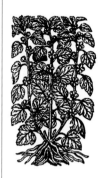

MEADOWSWEET

Filipendula ulmaria

Parts Used
Leaves, flower tops

We owe the word "aspirin" to the beautiful, aromatic meadowsweet.
During the Middle Ages, meadowsweet's delicate almond fragrance made it a popular air freshener, or "strewing herb."

In 1839, a German chemist discovered meadowsweet flower buds contained salicin. Salicin has powerful pain-relieving (analgesic), fever-reducing, and anti-inflammatory properties.

In 1853, German chemists working with an extract of meadowsweet synthesised acetylsalicylic acid. The new drug was named aspirin from the old botanical name for the herb (Spirea ulmaria).

In the late 1890s, a German chemist, became upset that his father's rheumatoid arthritis medication brought him so little relief. Hoffman worked at the Fredrich Bayer pharmaceutical company. He came upon the old reports of aspirin and prepared the drug.

Applications

HEADACHE, RHEUMATIC PAINS, FEVERISH COLDS, MUSCLES ACHES, DIGESTIVE UPSETS, CHILDHOOD DIARRHEOA

Infusion

Caution
Meadowsweet should not be given to children under age 2 or children under 16 suffering fevers from colds, flu, or chicken pox.

For a pleasantly astringent infusion, use 1 to 2 teaspoons of dried herb per cup of boiling water. Steep 10 minutes. Take for headaches, muscle aches, feverish colds, rheumatic pains and children's upset stomachs.

Tincture
Tinctures provide greater pain relief.

Compress
Soak a pad in a diluted tinctures and use on arthritic joints.

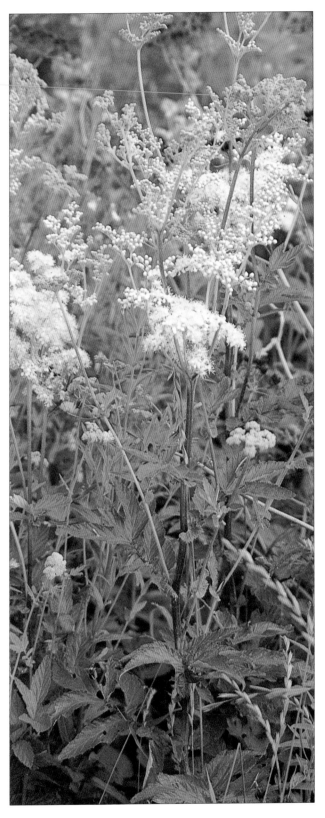

Meadowsweet is a perennial with stems that reach 60-180cm. It has elmlike leaves and large drooping clusters of small coiled white or pink flowers, which bloom throughout summer and have a fragrant, sweet almond aroma. It stands taller and has more striking flowers than most other meadow plants, hence its name queen-of-themeadow.

Meadowsweet does best in rich, moist, well-drained soil under partial shade. Harvest the leaves and flower tops when the plant is in bloom.

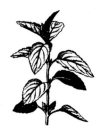

MINT

Mentha spp.

Parts used
Leaves, flower tops

All the mints were considered one plant until 1696, when British botanist John Ray differentiated them.
Mint was listed as a stomach soother in the Ebers Papyrus, the world's oldest surviving medical text.

Chinese and Ayurvedic physicians used mint as a tonic and digestive aid and as a treatment for colds, cough, and fever.

Contemporary herbalists recommend peppermint externally for itching and inflammations, and internally as a digestive aid and treatment for menstrual cramps, motion sickness, morning sickness, colds, cough, flu, congestion, headache, heartburn, fever, and insomnia. Of the two herbs peppermint is the more potent.

Applications

DIGESTIVE AID, DECONGESTANT, INFECTION PREVENTION, ITCHING, NAUSEA, INFLAMMED JOINTS, TRAVEL SICKNESS, WOUNDS

Essential oil
For wounds, burns and scalds apply a few drops of peppermint oil directly to the affected area.

A few drops of oil in water can be applied to the skin to relieve irritations and itching and to repell mosqitoes.

Inhalation
Put some fresh leaves in boiling water. Inhale to relieve nasal congestion.

Infusion
For a decongestant or digestive infusion, use 1 to 2 teaspoons of dried herb per cup of boiling water. Steep 10 minutes. Peppermint has a sharper taste than spearmint, and it cools the mouth.

Tincture

In a tincture, take quarter to 1 teaspoon up to three times a day.

In an herbal bath, fill a cloth bag with a few handfuls of dried or fresh herb and let the water run over it.

Caution

If mints cause minor discomforts, such as stomach upset or diarrheoa, use less or stop using it.

Because mint can irritate the mucous mebranes it should not be given to children for more than a week without a break.

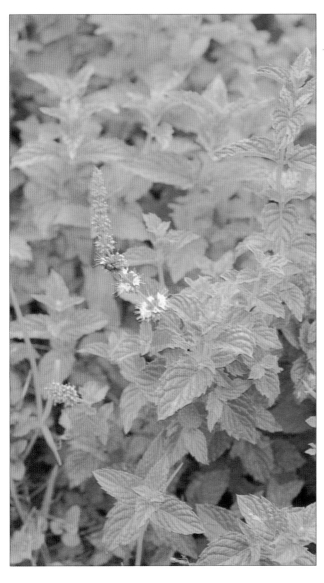

Spearmint and peppermint look alike, except peppermint grows taller, spreads by surface runners, has stems with a purplish cast, and has longer, less-wrinkled leaves.

Any piece of root with a joint or node can produce a plant. Contain your mint bed or plant in containers. In rich, moist, well-drained soil, under full sun or partial shade, spreading mints may become pests.

Frequent cutting encourages bushiness. Leaves may be harvested as they mature.

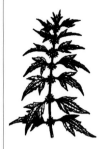

MOTHERWORT

Leonurus cardiaca

Parts used
Leaves, flowers, stems

The ancient Greeks and Romans used motherwort for both physical and emotional problems of the heart—palpitations and depression.

In ancient China, motherwort was reputed to promote longevity. In Europe, motherwort first became known as a treatment for cattle diseases.

Chines herbalists use the species mainly for menstrual disorders.

Applications

BLOOD PRESSURE, MENOPAUSAL SYNDROME, SORE EYES, TRANQUILLIZER

Infusion
For a tranquillizing, uterine stimulating, blood pressure-lowering infusion, use 1 to 2 teaspoons of dried herb per cup of boiling water. Steep 10 minutes. Drink up to 2 cups a day, a tablespoon at a time.

Also use as a tonic for menopausal syndrome and anxiety.

Motherwort tastes very bitter. Add sugar, honey, and lemon, or mix it into an herbal beverage tea to improve flavor.

Tincture
In a tincture, take half to 1 teaspoon up to twice a day.

Decoction
Use a weak decoction for conjunctivitis and tired eyes.

Caution
Avoid during pregnancy as motherwort stimulates the uterus.

Some people develop a rash from contact with this plant.

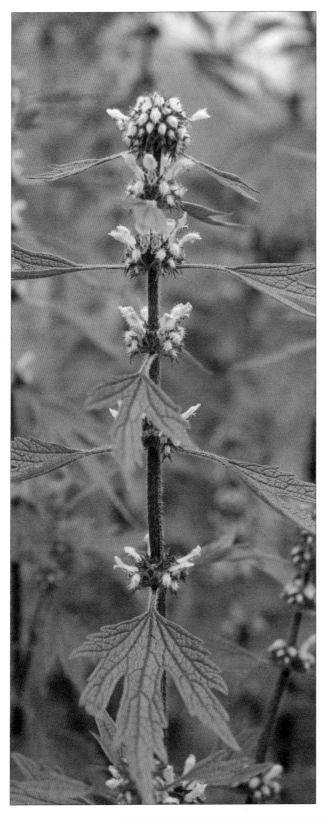

Motherwort's perennial root gives rise to stout, square stems tinged with red or violet, which grow to 120cm. Its lower leaves are sharply lobed, like maple. Its upper leaves are narrow and toothed. Motherwort produces whorls of small white, pink, or red flowers which bloom in summer.

Prefers rich, moist, well-drained soil and full sun but tolerates considerably less ideal conditions.

Harvest the entire plant after the flowers blossom.

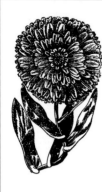

POT MARIGOLD

Calendula officinalis

Parts used
Petals

The ancients used marigold to "strengthen the heart" (Culpeper). It was also highly regarded for treating smallpox and measles.

In the 12th century it was believed that by looking at the plant would improve eyesight and clear the head.

The petals can be applied externally to help in a wide range of skin problems. Pot marigold is used today in many homeopathic remedies.

Applications

MENSTRUAL DISORDERS, INFLAMMATION, GASTRITIS, MOUTH ULCERS AND GUM PROBLEMS, SCALDS, SUNBURN, DRY SKIN, CHILBLAINS, ANXIETY, DRY ECZEMA, DIGESTION

Tincture
Take for menstrual disorders, especially period pain or irregular periods and for digestion.

Mouthwash
Use the infusion as a mouth wash to treat mouth ulcers or gum problems.

Infusion
Use the infusion for period pain, gastritis, or for menopausal problems.

Ointment
Apply to relieve dry skin, sunburn, scalds, inflammation of the skin or dry eczema.

Infused oil
Use for chilblains

Essential oil
5-10 drops of the oil added to a bath will relieve anxiety.

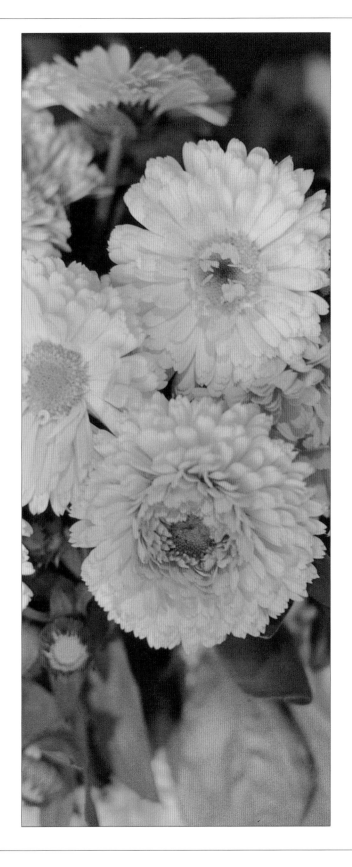

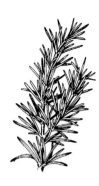

ROSEMARY

Rosmarinus officinalis

Parts used
Leaves

The ancients used rosemary as they used all aromatic, preservative herbs—for head, respiratory, and gastrointestinal problems. Traditional Chinese physicians mixed it with ginger and used it to treat headache, indigestion, insomnia, and malaria.

As recently as World War II, French nurses burned a mixture of rosemary leaves and juniper berries in hospital rooms as an antiseptic.

Contemporary herbalists say rosemary stimulates the circulatory, digestive, and nervous systems. They recommend it for headache, indigestion, depression, muscle pain, as a gargle to treat bad breath, externally to prevent premature baldness, and in baths for relaxation.

Applications

COLDS, RHEUMATIC PAINS, INDIGESTION, FATIGUE, SPRAINS, DANDRUFF

Infusion
For a pleasantly aromatic infusion to settle the stomach, clear a stuffed nose, relieve rheumatic pains or help indigestion use 1 teaspoon of crushed herb per cup of boiling water. Steep 10 to 15 minutes. Drink up to 3 cups a day.

Use as a final hair rinse to combat dandruff.

Tincture
In a tincture, use a quarter to half teaspoon up to three times a day.

Compress
Soak a pad in a hot infusion and use for sprains. Be sure to alternate with cold ice packs every two or three minutes.

Essential oil
A few drops in a hot bath will relieve aching limbs.

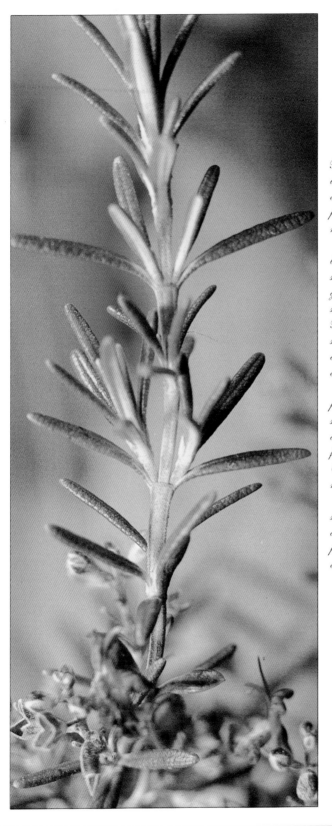

Rosemary is a woody, pine-scented, evergreen perennial with needlelike leaves.

Rosemary can be grown from seeds, but most herb growers prefer to start with cuttings. Plant cuttings in sandy soil, leaving only one-third of each twig showing.

Rosemary prefers light, sandy, well-drained soil and full sun. Overwatering may cause root rot.

Cut twigs and strip the leaves anytime after plants have become established.

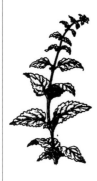

SKULLCAP

Scutellaria spp.

Parts used
Leaves

For centuries, Chinese physicians have used Asian skullcap *(S. baikalensis)* as a tranquilliz-er/sedative and treatment for convulsions.

Skullcap was first brought to the attention of physicians in the West in 1772 as a cure for rabies.

The herb was used primarily as a tranquill-iser/sedative for insomnia and nervousness, and for treatment of "intermittent fever" (malaria), convulsions, and delirium tremens of advanced alcoholism.

Contemporary herbalists recommend skullcap as a tranquillizer for insomnia, nervous tension, pre-menstrual syndrome, and drug and alcohol withdrawal.

Applications

TRANQUILLIZER, NERVOUS DISORDERS, INSOMNIA, PRE-MENSTRUAL TENSION

Infusion
For a tranquilising infusion, use 1 to 2 teaspoons of dried herb per cup boiling water. Steep 10 to 15 minutes. Drink up to three times a day for nervous exhaustion, over-anxiety and pre-menstrual tension.

Skullcap tastes bitter; adding honey, sugar, and lemon will make it palatable.

Tincture
Potent for calming the nerves.

Combine with lemon balm for nervous stress.

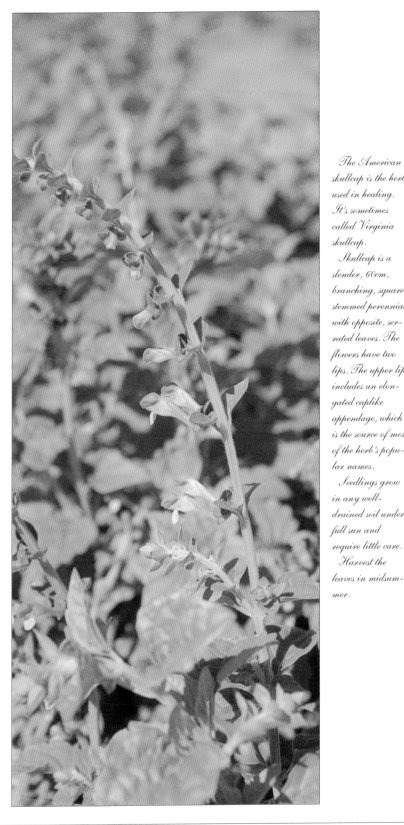

The American skullcap is the herb used in healing. It's sometimes called Virginia skullcap.

Skullcap is a slender, 60cm, branching, square-stemmed perennial with opposite, serrated leaves. The flowers have two lips. The upper lip includes an elongated caplike appendage, which is the source of most of the herb's popular names.

Seedlings grow in any well-drained soil under full sun and require little care.

Harvest the leaves in midsummer.

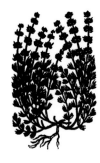

THYME

Thymus vulgaris

Parts used
Leaves, flower tops

The Romans also used thyme medicinally as a cough remedy, digestive aid, and treatment for intestinal worms.

As the centuries passed, it was used as an antiseptic during plagues, and those troubled by "melancholia" (depression) were advised to sleep on thyme-stuffed pillows.

By the late 17th century, apothecary shops were selling thyme oil as a topical antiseptic under the name oil of origanum.

From the mid-19th century through World War I, thyme enjoyed great popularity as an antiseptic.

Contemporary herbalists recommend thyme externally for wound disinfection and internally for indigestion, sore throat, laryngitis, cough, whooping cough, and nervousness.

Applications

SORE THROAT, COUGHS, CHEST INFECTION, UNSETTLED STOMACH, INSECT BITES, ANTISEPTIC

Infusion
For an infusion to help settle the stomach, soothe a cough, or possibly help relieve menstrual symptoms, use 2 teaspoons of dried herb per cup of boiling water. Steep 10 minutes. Drink up to 3 cups a day. Thyme tastes pleasantly aromatic with a faint clovelike aftertaste.

Gargle for a sore throat.

Tincture
In a tincture, take half to 1 teaspoon up to three times a day.

Once wounds have been thoroughly washed, apply a few drops of thyme tincture as an antiseptic.

Essential oil
Add 10 drops to 20ml water and apply to infected wounds and insect bites.

Caution
Thyme oil may cause a rash in sensitive individuals. Avoid therapeutic doses of thyme during pregnancy.

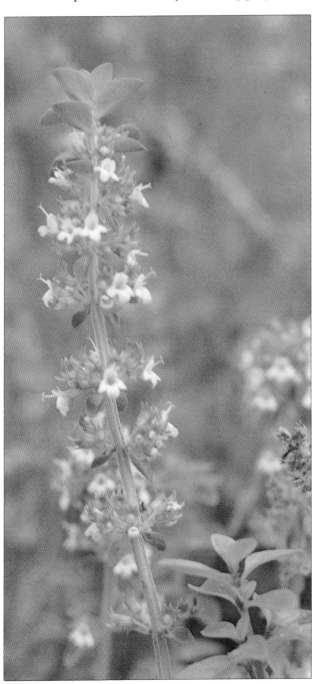

Thyme is an aromatic, perennial groundcover shrub that reaches about 30cm. It has small, virtually stalkless leaves and lilac or pink flowers that bloom in midsummer.

The best time for root division is in spring. Uproot a plant carefully, preserving as much of its root soil as possible. Divide it and replant the divisions 30cm apart in moist soil.

Once established, thyme requires little care. It prefers well-drained soil on the dry side.

Wetting thyme leaves during watering reduces their fragrance. Harvest the leaves and flower tops just before the flowers bloom. Dry and store them in airtight containers to preserve the herb's oil.

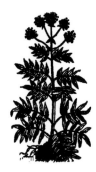

VALERIAN

Valeriana officinalis

Parts used
Rhizome, roots

Valerian has a disagreeable odor, and ancient Greek and Roman authorities called it fu. The term Valerian appeared around the 10th century, derived from the Latin valere, to be strong.

Dioscorides recommended valerian as a diuretic and antidote to poisons. Pliny considered it a pain reliever. Galen prescribed it as a decongestant. By the time the plant's name became valerian, early European herbalists considered it a panacea and also called it "All-heal".

During World War I, Europeans afflicted with "overwrought nerves" from artillery bombardment frequently took valerian.

All parts of valerian contain chemicals that have sedative properties known as valepotriates, but they occur in highest concentration in the roots.

Applications

TRANQUILLIZER, INSOMNIA, MUSCLE CRAMP, WOUNDS, ANXIETY, BLOOD PRESSURE

Infusion

Caution
Large amounts may cause headache, giddiness, blurred vision, restlessness, nausea, and morning grogginess.
Make sure you don't use for more than 2 weeks without a break.

For a potential sedative infusion anxiety and insomnia, use 2 teaspoons of powdered root per cup of water. Steep 10 to 15 minutes. Drink 1 cup before bed. Valerian tastes unpleasant. Add sugar, honey, and lemon.

Use on wounds and for drawing splinters.

Tincture
In a tincture, take half to 1 teaspoon before bed for insomnia.

Can be added to other herbs such as hyssop where anxiety has contributed to high blood pressure.

Compress
Soak a pad in the tincture and apply to muscles in cases of cramp.

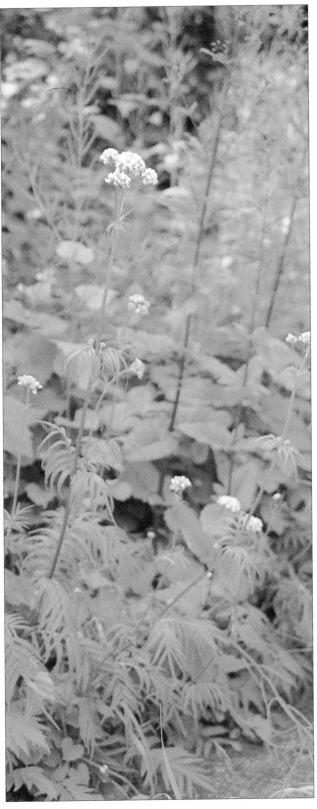

Medicinal valerian's roots consist of long, cylindrical fibres issuing from its rhizome.

Valerian leaves are fernlike. Tiny flowers— white, pink, or lavender—develop in umbrella-like clusters. When dried, valerian roots have an unpleasant odor.

Valerian grows in many soils, but does best in rich, moist, well-drained loam under full sun or partial shade. Once established, plants self-sow and spread by root runners.

Harvest roots in the autumn of their second year. Split thick roots to speed drying. Valerian's characteristic unpleasant odor develops as the roots dry.

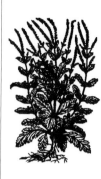

VERVAIN

Verbena officinalis

Parts used
Leaves, flowers, roots

Vervain acts like a mild aspirin, helping to relieve minor pains and inflammations.
The Romans spread vervain throughout Europe, where it became especially popular among the Druids, who used it in magic spells.

During the Middle Ages, vervain became a popular acne remedy. Those with pimples stood outside at night holding a handful of the herb wrapped in a cloth.

Contemporary herbalists recommend vervain as a tranquillizer, expectorant, menstruation promoter, and treatment for headache, fever, depression, seizures, wounds, dental cavities, and gum disease.

Applications

INFLAMMATION AND PAIN RELIEF, HEADACHE, NERVOUS TENSION, DEPRESSION, GUMS, INSOMNIA, BRUISES

Infusion
For a very bitter infusion using leaves and flowers to help treat headache, nervous tension, mild arthritis, and other minor pains, use 2 teaspoons of dried herb per cup of boiling water. Steep 10 to 15 minutes. Drink up to 3 cups a day. Mask vervain's bitterness with sugar, honey, and lemon.

Use as a mouthwash for ulcers and soft gums.

Tincture
In a tincture, use half to 1 teaspoon up to three times a day.

Take for nervous exhaustion and depression.

Poultice

Caution
Avoid during pregnancy.

Apply for insect bites, sprains and bruises

Ointment
Eczema and weeping sores.

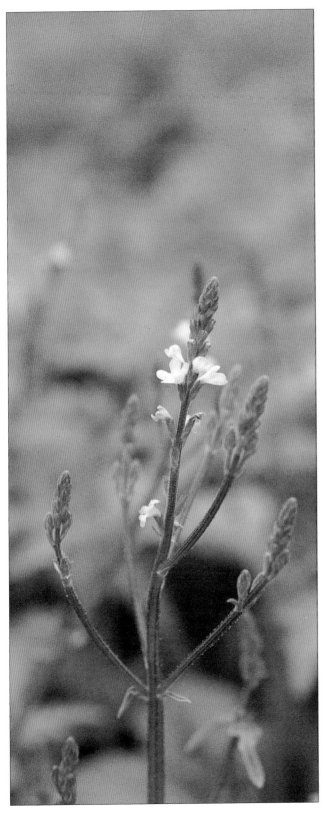

Vervain is a 180cm perennial with thin, erect, stiff stems. Its opposite leaves are oblong and toothed near the ground and lance-shaped and deeply lobed higher up. The plant develops slender flower spikes that bear small blue or lilac flowers. The herb's bluish flowers gave it the name blue vervain.

Although a perennial, this herb is short-lived; however, it self-sows. Vervain prefers rich, moist loam under full sun.

Harvest the leaves and flower tops as the plants flower.

YARROW

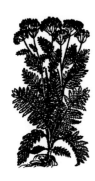

Achillea millefolium

Parts used
Leaves, stems, flower tops

Yarrow contains substances that help stop bleeding and have pain-relieving and anti-inflammatory properties helpful in wound treatment. It also is a digestive aid, menstrual remedy, and mild sedative.

Dioscorides, a physician attached to Roman legions, recommended rubbing the crushed plant on wounds.

Contemporary herbalists recommend yarrow as "an herbal Band-Aid" and prescribe it for fevers, urinary tract infections, and as a digestive aid.

Applications

WOUNDS, DIGESTIVE AID, MENSTRUAL CRAMPS, NOSE BLEED, HAY FEVER,

Infusion
For a tranquillizing infusion to help aid digestion or help treat menstrual cramps, use 1 to 2 teaspoons of dried herb per cup of boiling water. Steep 10 to 15 minutes. Drink up to 3 cups a day. Yarrow tastes tangy and bitter with some astringency. To improve flavor, add honey, sugar, or lemon.

To help promote healing, apply it externally to clean wounds, inflammations and eczema.

Inhalation
Use fresh leaves in boiling water for hay fever and mild asthma.

Leaves
Stop a nose bleed by inserting a leaf in the nostril. Press fresh leaves and flower tops into cuts before washing and bandaging them.

Caution
Avoid during pregnancy. High doses can turn urine dark brown. Do not be alarmed.

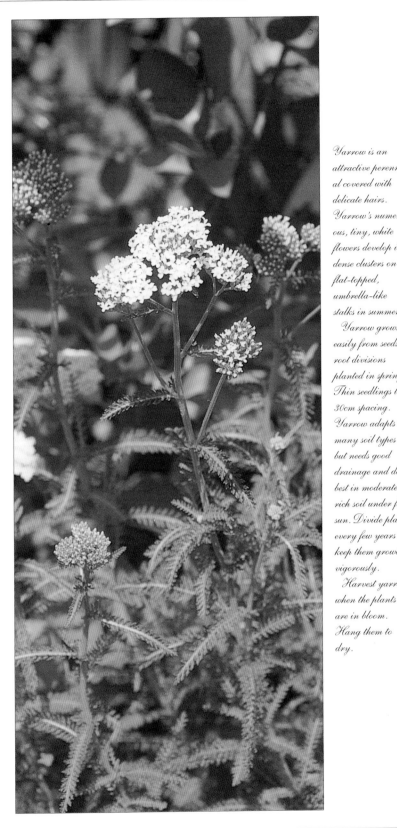

Yarrow is an attractive perennial covered with delicate hairs. Yarrow's numerous, tiny, white flowers develop in dense clusters on flat-topped, umbrella-like stalks in summer.

Yarrow grows easily from seeds or root divisions planted in spring. Thin seedlings to 30cm spacing. Yarrow adapts to many soil types but needs good drainage and does best in moderately rich soil under full sun. Divide plants every few years to keep them growing vigorously.

Harvest yarrow when the plants are in bloom. Hang them to dry.

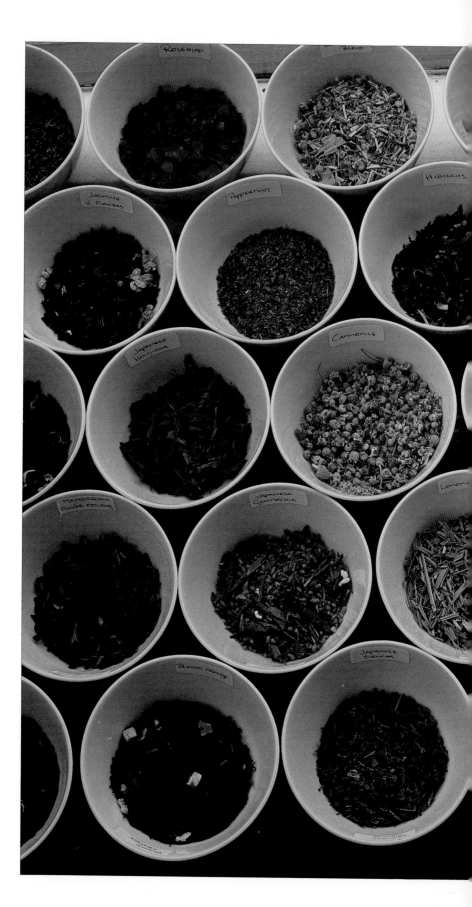

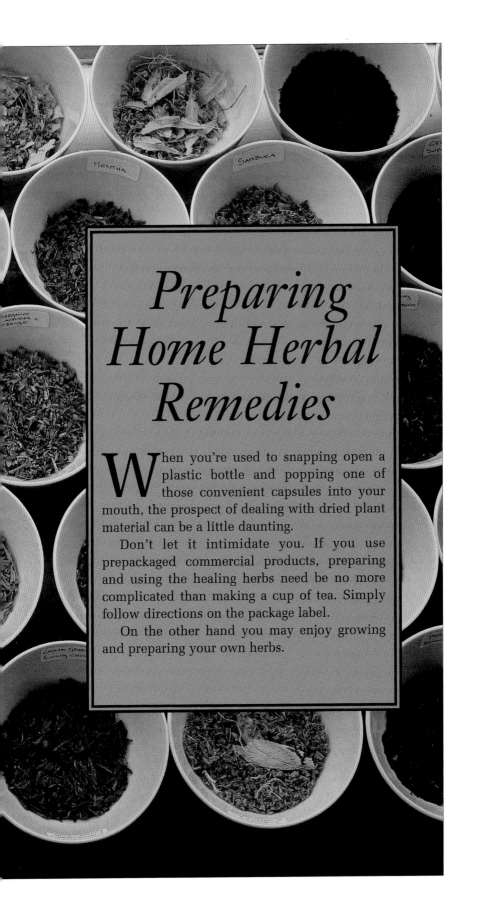

Preparing Home Herbal Remedies

When you're used to snapping open a plastic bottle and popping one of those convenient capsules into your mouth, the prospect of dealing with dried plant material can be a little daunting.

Don't let it intimidate you. If you use prepackaged commercial products, preparing and using the healing herbs need be no more complicated than making a cup of tea. Simply follow directions on the package label.

On the other hand you may enjoy growing and preparing your own herbs.

Drying

Healing herb formulas almost always begin with dried plant material, so fresh herbs, should be dried before they're stored or used.

Traditionally, most herbs were simply hung in a warm, dry, shady spot until they crumbled easily. Roots were washed, split, and spread in a single layer on a clean surface. Traditional drying methods are still used today. In fact, some herb shops sell herbs in dried bunches.

But traditional drying has two disadvantages. It often requires more room than most of us have, and it takes time. To preserve the aromatic volatile oils in many herbs, the faster the drying time, the better.

At home you can place herbs on a sheet of foil in a 35 degree C oven. Many ovens, however, don't heat evenly, so some plant material might char while the rest remains too moist.

Crushing

Most dry herbs are powdered to reduce them to a convenient form to use. The mortar and pestle still works well for those who process only small amounts of herbs.

Storing

Light and oxygen are the two biggest destroyers of herb flavour and medicinal potency.

Store medicinal herbs in opaque glass or ceramic containers. Fill them to the top. As you use the herbs, add cotton wool to the containers to limit the amount of oxygen inside.

When stored properly, aromatic herbs can remain good for more than a year, and non-aromatic herbs much longer.

Moisture is another problem. If your herbs get wet, redry them quickly to prevent mold.

Insects also take their toll. Drying kills many pests, but watch for signs of infestation.

Preparation

Infusions

Infusions are extracts made from medicinal herbs using their flowers, leaves, and stems. Infusions are

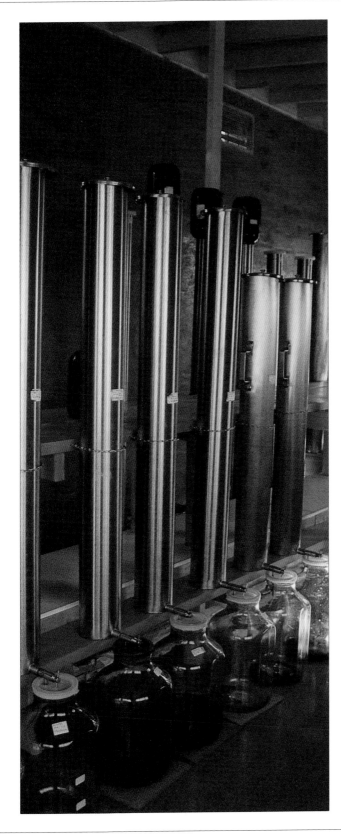

Tinctures being pre-pared

not teas. They are prepared like teas, but they are steeped longer to become stronger.

The standard traditional infusion recipe calls for 30g of dried herb steeped in a 500ml of boiling water for 10 to 20 minutes.

Infusions do not have a long shelf life. They should be made as needed, so many of today's herbalists recommend half to 1 rounded teaspoon per cup of boiling water steeped for the same amount of time.

You can use fresh herbs instead of dried to make an infusion by simply doubling the amount of herb.

Decoctions

Decoctions are extracts made from roots and barks. The active chemicals in roots and barks are more difficult to extract, so instead of steeping, you gently simmer the dried herb material in boiling water for 10 to 20 minutes.

Making a Tincture

Tinctures are extracts made with alcohol rather than water. They are highly concentrated, so they're more portable. They also remain potent longer.

Use 100 proof vodka or brandy. The standard tincture recipe calls for 30g of crushed, dried herb steeped in 140g of distilled spirits for six weeks.

Some tips

• Shake the mixture every few days to encourage alcohol uptake of the herb's medicinal constituents.
• As tinctures develop, the liquid level may go down. Top up with distilled spirits.
• After six weeks you can strain out the plant material, but it's not necessary.

Those who do not drink alcohol can make tinctures using warm vinegar. Herbalists recommend wine or apple cider vinegar, not the white variety. The directions are the same.

Capsules

Powdered herbs can also be packed inside standard gelatin capsules.

If you make capsules, measure how much powdered herb fits into the capsules you're using so you won't exceed the dosage recommended.

Index

L

Laringitis 50
Lemon balm 12
Liver 11
Longevity 42

M

Malaria 48
Marshmallow 36
Meadowsweet 38
Menstrual irregulari-
ties 11 20 26 28
40 42 48 50 54 56
Migraine headache
30
Milk (breast) promot-
er 28
Minor fractures 24
Mint 40
Morning sickness 34
40
Motherwort 42
Motion sickness 34
40
Mouth inflamma-
tions 20
Mouth ulcers 54
Muscle ache 38 46
cramp 52
damage 22

N

Nausea 34 40
Nervousness 48 50
56
Nervous stomach 28
Nosebleed 56

O

Obesity 18 26

P

Pain relief 54 56
Palpitation 42
Period pain 28
Pneumonia 26
Pot Marigold 24

R

Respiratory ailments
11 36
Rheumatic pain 38
46
Rosemary 46

S

Scalds 10 40
Sciatica 16
Scrapes 10 21 36
Skin infections and
disorders 16 32
Skullcap 48
Sores 12 16
Sore throat 28 36
50
Sprains 22 46
Storing herbs 60
Strained eyes 20 21
Stress 20
Sunburn 10
Swellings 12
Swollen feet 26

T

Tension 12 20 48
Thyme 50
Tinctures 61
Tranquillisers 42 48
52 54
Travel sickness 40

U

Ulcers 16 26
Urinary tract infec-
tion 16 18
Urine production 26

V

Valerian 52
Vervain 54

W

Warts 26 32
Weight loss 26
Whooping cough 50
Worms 50
Wounds 10 22 36
40 50 51 52 54 56

Y

Yarrow 56